D1125143

Caregiver Stress
Neurobiology to the Rescue

By Heidi Crockett, LCSW

May you fill in the blanks and transform your fall

- Heidi Crockett

Caregiver Stress: Neurobiology to the Rescue

Copyright © 2015 Heidi Crockett

All rights reserved. No part of this book may be reproduced in any form or by any electronic or mechanical means, including information storage and retrieval systems, without permission in writing from the author. For information, contact HeidiCrockett@gmail.com.

The content of this book is for general instruction only. Each person's physical, mental, and emotional condition is unique. The instruction in this book is not intended to replace or interrupt the reader's relationship with a physician or other professional. Please consult your doctor for matters pertaining to your specific health.

To contact the author, visit

www.HeidiCrockett.com

ISBN: 0996232206
ISBN-13: 978-0-9962322-0-3

Dynamic Learning
314 Shore Dr. E.
Oldsmar, FL 34677-3916

Published in the United States by Dynamic Learning

DEDICATION

To Roger

Thank you for teaching me about death
and what it means to live.

CONTENTS

ACKNOWLEDGMENTS

I first learned about interpersonal neurobiology through my Professor, Stephanie Swann, at the University of Georgia. I want to thank her for this introduction to the subject, and also Dr. Daniel Siegel for his tremendous research. Lastly, I want to thank my late husband, Roger Millen, for being the inspiration for this book and for teaching me everything I know about caregiving.

1 INTRODUCTION

Many of us have to act as caregivers to our loved ones, family members or friends on a daily basis; this role is vital, but can take a serious toll over time. The stress that caregivers face day after day has a long-term impact on their health. Recent advances in neurobiology show how we can use our mind to reshape our brain to better handle stress. Thus, it is crucial for caregivers to understand neurobiology and how it can be used to better manage stress.

A 2013 Alzheimer's Association publication says that "it is high stress, not caregiving *per se*, that increases the risk of mortality."[i] In other words, learning how to manage stress is vital for your long-term health as a caregiver.

This book is an educational toolkit for caregivers.

I apply concepts from interpersonal neurobiology in a workbook format while interspersing my experiences as a caregiver. I hope that it inspires self-reflection and insight, so you can better digest and transform stress.

2 YOUR CAREGIVING JOURNEY

"Men fear death, as if unquestionably the greatest evil, and yet no man knows that it may not be the greatest good."
—William Mitford

Imagine you are falling from the sky without a parachute. You are falling at 120 mph. What are your thoughts and feelings as you fall? Are you terrified, exhilarated, or in awe? Does your life flash before your very eyes?

Caregiving is a lot like falling out of the sky at 120 mph. No matter how many books you've read or support groups you've been to, the extreme emotions evoked by caregiving are yours alone as you fall. If you are the primary caregiver, it is *you* in charge of your loved one, 24 hours a day, seven days a week.

According to dream interpretation, things that

appear "bad" in the dream world can actually be "good." One example is falling. Normally if you were falling through the sky you would be dead when you hit the ground. Fortunately *in your dream* all kinds of things can happen as you fall—you can wake yourself up, you can start to fly, or you can hit the ground and start walking with no problem. In dream interpretation, being awake in the dream and willing to let yourself "die," turning the falling into flying, or finishing falling and keeping the dream going represent forms of transformation or rebirth. One goal of this workbook is for you to experience and write about transformation along your caregiving journey. Another goal is that you are able to witness yourself "falling" as you experience extreme stress and that you feel curious and open as opposed to terrified.

You might be wondering, "How can we get there?" Or, "Why should we put in the effort to get there?" Or, "Why is the author writing about falling and dreams, I thought this book was about neurobiology!" I promise to answer these questions systematically throughout the book. First, we'll begin with what the research says about caregiver stress and its effects on your long-term health...after you answer some questions about falling.

As a caregiver, when do you feel most out-of-control? _____

_____

_____

What parts of caregiving give you the most anxiety?

_____

_____

_____

Do the experiences that you just wrote about make you feel like you are falling through the sky without a parachute? Why or why not? _____

_____

_____

_____

_____

Are you willing to invest time and energy to cultivate an open and curious attitude when "falling"? State why or why not: _____

_____

_____

3 THE EFFECTS OF CAREGIVER STRESS

Roger and I sat facing each other at the dinner table. We were having yet another conversation about his dreaded future.   It was February of 2009, just five months before he would pass away.

"I'm dying," he said in an anxious and urgent tone.

"You're dying," I replied, looking into his eyes and taking his hand.

He had a grade IV glioblastoma since October of 2006 and had undergone two brain surgeries. Glioblastoma is the most malignant and aggressive type of brain tumor, with most patients surviving just over one year, even with the best available treatment. Periodically and repetitively Roger would revisit the subject of his death because it caused him *great* anxiety.

We looked at each other.   We had been through

conversations similar to this one so many times before that I was left without words this time. What more could I *possibly* say to him? What can anyone say to soothe someone who has a terminal diagnosis but doesn't want to die? It was a hard place to be for both of us. We were stuck.

Roger's cancer journey taught me about death and what it means to be alive. In the beginning, I would notice my body tensing when his fear and anxiety about dying arose. We spent *insane* amounts of time in the denial stage. We were constantly researching new cancer treatments and diets, then endlessly preparing food and ordering supplements.

I still remember the look of pure sympathy and knowing that came from the manager at the Tree of Life Center in Patagonia, AZ, on the afternoon before I left to return home after a two week visit. I told him that my husband and I were thinking about relocating so he could be on the raw food diet and he told me how his wife had died of breast cancer and how like us they had searched frantically for alternative solutions. I told him that I'd decided moving to Arizona wouldn't be a good fit for us as we needed to keep our social support network and close access to good doctors. He gave me such a look of compassion and understanding that I will never forget.

Being a caregiver is not about having the answers, it's about loving someone and trying. It's about doing your best, giving it your all, and about what happens when you go past your breaking point in that effort.

Looking back, my heart would break into a million, tiny pieces *each time* Roger said he was dying with that sense of urgency and anxiety in his voice. I didn't want him to die. Of course I didn't want him to die! I felt powerless and sad when he would say it. Besides my feeling reaction to his words and circumstances, as his caregiver, I felt like I must perfectly address his feelings and needs at the same time. It was an impossible task, and yet, the futility of the situation helped me break through to new ways of knowing and experiencing life.

Caregiving means we live in circumstances we often *don't want* and with a convergence of intense, conflicting emotions. Living in such a state has effects on the body and the brain.

Many studies on caregivers show, "prolonged exposure to the chronic stress of caregiving...

predispose caregivers to hypertension and cardiovascular disease."[ii]   In other words, you are more likely to develop hypertension and/or high blood pressure if you are a caregiver.

Caregiving leads to increased stress.   This is probably the very reason why you are reading this book right now…maybe you're wondering what you can do about the overwhelming feelings you're grappling with as a caregiver? Perhaps you hope that gaining more information will comfort and calm your spirit.

Like the quote says at the start of chapter one, you may begin your caregiving journey thinking that you know clearly what is "good" and "evil," *but do you?* Certainly in the beginning, I thought that Roger's brain tumor diagnosis was the worst thing **EVER**.   Over time, I learned that if we can open into a state of unknowing, there is a sacredness in the space between what we think we know about reality and what we ultimately come to know *as we fall.*

From this perspective, we can begin to ask ourselves curious questions about falling instead of immediately assuming it is bad.   One clear example of not knowing what's "good" or "bad" is that this book wouldn't exist unless Roger had had his cancer diagnosis. In this sense, the gifts he gave me while living live on through the interconnectedness of my sharing this book with you and your experience as a caregiver.

This book is intended to provide you with useful information, especially tips for dealing with stress. We'll begin by defining interpersonal neurobiology and optimal mental health in the next chapter. Using the Wellness Triangle, we'll learn that while some effects of stress are inevitable, most can be *redirected* in healthy ways. One metaphor for this redirection is *transforming the outcome of your dream* as mentioned in chapter one. There are writing exercises throughout the book: these are for you to better understand the material and make it relevant to your current circumstances. Moreover, these reflective activities are intended to be like seeds which you can cultivate to transform the outcome of your life as a caregiver, as if you were in the falling dream I just mentioned.

4 OPTIMAL MENTAL HEALTH

"May I learn to see with the eyes of understanding and love. May I learn to see and touch the seeds of joy and happiness in myself and others. May I learn to identify the sources of anger, craving, delusion and anxiety and may I choose based on my higher self when faced with cravings." --Buddhist prayer of loving-kindness

The sun was setting as I rode along in my friend's black car. We were going fast on the interstate, as fast as everyone else, when suddenly the car started shaking. Something was very wrong. My friend, Ben, immediately pulled over onto the median. He stepped outside and sure enough, the rear driver's side tire was flat. We had about fifteen minutes before dark and cars continued to zip by at dangerous speeds. I stood in awe as he went into action, first opening the trunk and locating the spare, then sitting by the tire just a few feet away from cars zooming by at 80 plus miles per hour.

Like clockwork, he used the socket wrench to remove the flat tire's bolts and quickly changed the tire. If it had turned dark, the situation would have become even more dangerous with him sitting outside in the dark on the median and us having no flashlight. Another issue was the steep ditch just to our right, which prevented us from moving the car any further away from the highway.

This scenario highlights the optimal mental functioning that Ben demonstrated in those 20 minutes. His body sensed the wind and noise created by the cars whizzing past. He experienced fear for his life and anxiety as daylight was slipping away. Nevertheless, he was able to focus on one activity and shelve his emotions. As we got back in the car to drive to our destination, both of us let out audible sighs of relief.

Caregivers live with a similar sense of urgency and danger as Ben had that day. Unfortunately, we do not have one isolated, stressful event to tend to, but rather a pile of stress like an endlessly high stack of plates at a buffet table. That's why I described caregiving like "falling without a parachute from the sky" earlier. If you have been a caregiver for any significant amount of time, the stress piles so high that we know the stack of plates **will** fall. It **has** to fall. It must, as we are only human. In this book I will try to demonstrate that the problem isn't so much the fact that we fall, but our attitude when and after we hit the ground. Sometimes over and over again.

Ben's optimal functioning came from good mental health in the moment, but also from his prior wisdom and experience. Obviously that wasn't the first time Ben had changed a car tire. Some questions in this book will ask you to think about your own prior experiences, so you can harness your wisdom from the past and bring it into your current circumstances.

Also, we forget that it wasn't only Ben who suffered stress that day: I was there watching, feeling anxious and powerless. Caregivers forget that even if they are not directly experiencing the more severe symptoms of the person they are caring for, that the experience of caregiving impacts their health.

So, while falling is inevitable on your caregiving journey…whether it's your best china plates or falling from the sky…interpersonal neurobiology can teach us how to fall gracefully, or even how to fly.

Dr. Dan Siegel writes, *"Interpersonal neurobiology is not a branch of neuroscience—it is not the same, for example, as social neuroscience. Instead, this field is an open forum for all ways of knowing to collaborate in deepening and expanding our way of understanding reality, the human mind, and well-being."*[iii] In another article he writes, *"Interpersonal neurobiology attempts to extract the wisdom from more than a dozen different disciplines of science to weave a picture of human experience and the process of change across the lifespan."*[iv] The goal of this book is to extract some of the complex wisdom derived from neurobiology[v] and simplify it for caregivers to use. It is meant as only your starting place on a diverse, multifaceted subject.

This book uses neurobiology to define optimal mental health; before we start, think about your definition. Take a moment and write down some adjectives that describe an optimal mental state:_____

_____

_____

Recall a moment in your life when you felt you were coming from a good mental state. Describe how you felt and what you did:_____

_____

_____

_____

_____

What is your definition of optimal mental health?

_____

_____

_____

_____

_____

I define optimal mental health using the "Triangle of Well-Being" developed by UCLA neurobiologist Dan Siegel. I refer to this as the "Wellness Triangle" throughout the book. The three tips of the Wellness Triangle merge into one unit of optimal functioning: all three points are equally important and will be examined more closely as we proceed through this book.

Wellness Triangle

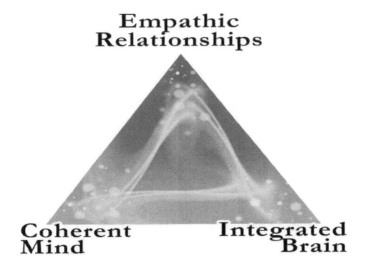

Empathic Relationships

Coherent Mind

Integrated Brain

According to the "Wellness Triangle" theory, to have "optimal mental health," all three tips of the triangle should be optimally functioning so that **you have three points of balance and quality** in your relationships, your mind and your brain:

- in your real-world empathic **relationships**
- in your relationship with your **mind** and thoughts
- in the physical integration between and inside the different parts of your **brain**[vi]

Before reading further, take a moment and think about how you fit in with the Wellness Triangle.

Name an example of a relationship that makes you feel connected. Write about what you think is most helpful about it:_____

_____

_____

_____

Name an example of a relationship that makes you feel unloved and without balance and quality in that relationship:_____

_____

_____

_____

On a scale of one to ten, with ten being the best, think about all your relationships which serve as your social support system when you are under stress. What number would you give yourself on the empathic relationships tip of the Wellness Triangle? Why that number? _____

_____

_____

_____

Name an example of a situation when your thoughts feel scattered. When do you typically not have balance and quality in your mind?_____

_____

_____

_____

_____

Name an example of a situation when your thoughts feel more coherent and collected. Write about when you have balance in your mind:_____

_____

_____

_____

_____

On a scale of one to ten, think about the quality of your own mind. Can you use it to hold attention and to come up with a game plan about how to soothe yourself when under stress? What number would you give yourself on the coherent mind tip of the Wellness Triangle? Why that number?_____

_____

_____

_____

We will be answering questions about your brain integration tip of the triangle later. First, we'll focus on relationships as we journey around the Wellness Triangle, one point at a time.

5 EMPATHIC RELATIONSHIPS TIP

"It would be difficult to overestimate the importance of human relationships. If love does not make the world go around, then surely relationships do. In the world of the personal, the world of work, and the world at large, relationships between people are a critical and decisive force."[vii] –Roberta M. Gilbert, M.D.

When someone gives us their time, presence, love and attention, it is like nourishment to our mental health and to our soul. High-quality empathic relationships occur when we feel that we have received the loving presence and attention of another person: they are VITAL to our mental health. Studies show that recipients of affectionate communication are at less risk of physical illness and have a greater ability to heal from the effects of illness or injuries.[viii] In other words, *high-quality interpersonal interactions are healing to the body.*

Wellness Triangle

Empathic
Relationships

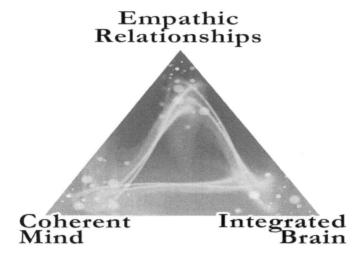

Coherent
Mind

Integrated
Brain

EMPATHIC RELATIONSHIPS

Think about all your relationships with friends, with family, with people you love and who love you. Write the names of these people (from the past and present) here:_____

_____

_____

_____

_____

Cultivate gratitude for having these folks in your life. Write what you most appreciate about them:_____

_____

_____

_____

_____

_____

_____

Stella Resnick PhD, a well-known researcher on the subject of love, writes that during intimacy, "your hearts are entrained and actually begin to beat in rhythm."[xi] Next, the hormonal, immune, and respiratory systems align. *Countless* benefits such as decreased anger, anxiety, and depression occur with increased intimacy and connection. Positive health benefits result both from sexual and non-sexual forms of intimacy. Examples of non-sexual intimacy include an intellectually stimulating conversation over a cup of coffee or reading a bedtime story to a beloved child or grandchild.

If you used to be in a reciprocal relationship with your spouse but it is now primarily a caregiving relationship, remember how important it is to find these nourishing "foods" of affectionate communication and intimacy. Be sure that you are "filling in" the gaps of what you have lost either by strengthening existing connections with friends and family and/or making new connections. In social work, the general term for these high-quality, interpersonal relationships is your "social support network." The same advice goes with this term: those who have a good social support network fare better when they are besieged by stressful circumstances.

Think about a relationship that isn't meeting your needs. Think about one person here: _____

Do you have the ability to set boundaries, say "no," or otherwise distance yourself from this person? What is most difficult about this person?_____

_____

_____

Name some more difficult people in your life:

_____

_____

What is hard about being around these people?_____

_____

_____

_____

Make of list of things you can do that would make it easier to say "no":_____

_____

_____

What small thing can you commit to doing out of the above list?_____

_____

_____

It goes without saying that the person you are caregiving is probably the hardest person to say "no" to and set healthy boundaries (especially if their condition deteriorates). Everyone's needs are different. Don't compare yourself to others. When I was caregiving my husband Roger, I reached the point of breakdown and had to move out of my home for two months and hire a live-in caregiver. I took care of my husband for eight hours each day and then retreated to my rented room two blocks away. I moved through intense feelings of guilt and failure during that time, but I did what I had to do for myself (See "Affirmations for Caregivers" at the end of the book. Saying aloud or thinking those affirmations, especially the ones in bold, served to comfort and strengthen my spirit).

Caregiving Roger was the hardest thing I have ever done. Like many caregivers, I sustained an injury (my right wrist), and didn't seek medical attention until after he passed away. You must try to do your best to care for yourself and ask for help, over and over, even when others say "no" and you feel uncomfortable asking.

Practice making and strengthening your interpersonal relationships at the time when you most need them. Now is when you find out who are truly your friends. If you feel alone and isolated, join a local support group. Reach out and connect. Someone else may need to hear exactly what you are going through.

Write about one way that you have not been taking care of yourself:_____

_____

_____

Can you commit to doing something about it? First make a list of all the different activities you have done in the past that you consider self-care:_____

_____

_____

_____

Looking at that list, write out what you are currently

doing to take care of you:_____

_____

_____

_____

Name something small that you can commit to doing to better take care of you:_____

_____

_____

Reflecting on your answers, write about what you are going to do to strengthen your relationships (e.g., contact a friend that you haven't spoken to in a long while, join a support group, etc.):_____

_____

_____

Draw a picture of   Draw a picture of
yourself stressed out: yourself at peace:

How did it feel to draw those pictures?_____

_____

Which person are you more of the time?_____

_____

Do you wish your above answer was different? If yes, how could it be different? _____

_____

6 USING HUMOR

"The human phenomenon is serious and tragic, but at the very same time, there is a comical or humorous aspect to most serious situations." —Murray Bowen

Stu and I had dropped Roger off at the urologist's office and rushed to the health food store to buy groceries. Stu was a dear friend: we had both been students at the Florida School of Massage in Gainesville, Florida. At first he had been a roommate, then when I started having a mental breakdown, he had graciously agreed to work eight hours a day as a live-in caregiver to avoid having to move Roger to a nursing home.

"You don't know what a Jakfruit is???! Oh my God, you are STUUUUUU-pid!" I said this to Stu in an unusually loud voice at the health food store. We simultaneously burst into uncontrollable laughter.

"I'm not STUPID, you're STUPID! Eat s*** and die!" Stu replied, ("Eat s*** and die" was an inside joke). We burst into maniacal laughter.

Suddenly it was as if the mini-stage we'd created was broken and we realized we were not alone in the store. We looked at each other knowing that we had been uncharacteristically socially inappropriate with our outburst. We both shrugged our shoulders and continued shopping. *We knew we needed that laughter to survive.*

If I only had two things to take as tools with me on the treacherous journey of caregiving, I would pick prayer and laughter. (Prayer is discussed later in the chapter on optimal spiritual health.)

Write about something funny in your caregiving journey. Try to write the whole story if you can remember it:_____

_____

_____

_____

_____

_____

_____

_____

_____

_____

Is there another funny story that you can think of but you don't want to write or say it because it might seem socially inappropriate? Go ahead! Write about it anyway, (you never know when you might want to remember a funny story and here you have a chance to write down all the details before you forget): _____

_____

_____

_____

_____

_____

_____

_____

_____

_____

_____

_____

_____

_____

_____

_____

_____

_____

_____

What can you do to bring more humor into your life?_____

_____

_____

Stu and I used to watch those Saturday Night Live Digital Shorts (warning explicit) or Strindberg & Helium videos.[xii]   Another suggestion is searching "Laughter Yoga" videos online and *doing the exercises, (don't just watch the video)*.

As you think and talk about your funny experiences, the caregiving scenes you describe might *seem like* you are making fun of your loved one. *Try to remember that they would want you happy and laughing.*   You are not laughing at them, but with them in your connected hearts. Sometimes when you're falling, all you can do is laugh or cry. And laughing is definitely more fun.

7 COHERENT MIND TIP

"One of the key practical lessons of modern neuroscience is that the power to direct our attention has within it the power to shape our brain's firing patterns, as well as the power to shape the architecture of the brain itself." —Daniel J. Siegel, M.D.

This chapter will explore the coherent mind tip of the Wellness Triangle. Dr. Siegel defines the mind as "the process that regulates the flow of information and energy."[xiii] I use the term "mind" to refer to the part of your awareness that is able to focus attention. A coherent mind can comfortably focus attention for long periods of time. It is able to change focus suddenly when required but can stay attentive before, after, and during the change.

Think about Ben's mind when he changed that flat tire. He was focused and calm, but as I discovered in the car ride after, he also had feelings of fear which he noticed but put aside for the more important task at hand. A coherent mind can shelve emotions lovingly.

In an upcoming chapter on brain integration, we go into what happens in the brain when it's stressed. We'll learn how stress can interfere with the mind's capacity to hold attention. Meanwhile, this chapter discusses what is possible with the mind.

Well-known mindfulness research performed by Jon Kabat-Zinn shows that 45 minutes of daily meditation for 6 weeks causes permanent, positive changes in the brain.[xiv] Dr. Siegel quotes this research saying: "*Recent studies of mindful awareness practices reveal that it can result in profound improvements in a range of physiological, mental, and interpersonal domains. Cardiac, endocrine, and immune functions are improved with mindful practices.*"[xv]

I like the way that Dr. Siegel introduces the idea of meditation. He writes, "*I introduce meditation to patients frequently now. Because I don't have a big background in meditation, I don't feel like I'm a religious zealot because I'm just offering this form of mental training because I think it is a part of brain hygiene. This is literally what I tell my patients: 'I'm going to teach you a technique that is a form of brain hygiene. You brush your teeth every day, right? This is a way of brushing your brain every day.' And I also say it's a form of mental floss. You know, you're getting the garbage out between the different synapses, loosening the hardening of our categories. Maybe it's simpler if we just leave the image as simply brushing your brain. Mindful awareness expands our sense of self by dissolving the prison of repeating patterns of thought and response."*[xvi]

If this is interesting to you, consider investing some time in meditation in order to cultivate the coherent mind tip. Even 15 minutes a day can make a big difference.

Next is the Wellness Triangle diagram with some questions to reflect on the quality of your mind.

Wellness Triangle

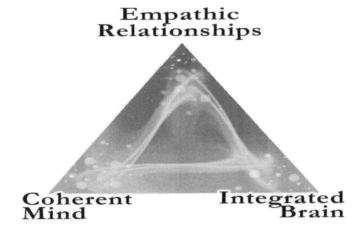

Empathic
Relationships

Coherent
Mind

Integrated
Brain

COHERENT MIND

What do you think about what you just read on the power of meditation (like its capacity improve cardiac or immune function)?_____

_____

_____

_____

Have you meditated before? What is your experience with mindful awareness practices including pranayama, connected breathing, Tai Chi, Qigong, and/or Gentle Yoga?_____

_____

_____

_____

Do you frequently have thoughts and/or words *racing* in your brain? What is your relationship with your thoughts?_____

_____

_____

_____

What activities help decrease racing thoughts?

_____

_____

_____

Can you commit to doing one new activity in the next seven days? (For ideas, health food stores often have a free Natural Awakenings magazine with local events.)_____

What activities do you do to help balance and ground you?_____

_____

_____

What can you do to calm your central nervous system when you are experiencing increased anxiety?

_____

_____

_____

How you answer this question about calming the nervous system is at the crux of learning how to manage caregiver stress in healthy ways. An excellent evidence-based book which comes with a CD with guided meditations is "The Mindful Way through Depression: Freeing Yourself from Chronic Unhappiness."[xvii] Jon Kabat-Zinn is one of the authors and it is not just helpful for people with depression, but rather a great book for anyone who wants to explore mindfulness to relieve stress.

Other activities that strengthen the coherent mind tip are exercise, a good night's sleep, and adequate hydration. They are essential building blocks to creating a calm mind. A thought-provoking book for those curious about sleep time or experiencing insomnia is "Hush: A Book of Bedtime Contemplations." Next are two quotes from this book.

"From the perspective of waking, falling asleep is an accident. Sleep is the slippery, downhill side of the day. We cannot intentionally go there. We can only slip, slide or fall into it. We slip out of waking and fall—which is suggestive of an accident—asleep. Evening rest and relaxation make us accident prone."

What do you like about this quote?_____

_____

_____

_____

How is the use of the word falling here similar or different than falling through the sky or falling china plates?_____

_____

_____

_____

"Going to bed with the same waking mindset
we sported all day is like sleeping in our clothes.
Though most of us routinely change our clothes before bed, few of
us effectively change our minds. We unthinkingly smuggle daytime
waking ways of being into night's domain of sleep and dreams.
Waking life is driven primarily by intention while night
consciousness is primarily informed by receptivity. We know how
to change our minds. We do it all the time. We simply need to
remember and be willing to do so at bedtime."[xxviii]

What do you like about this quote?_____

_____

_____

What is your attitude and approach to sleep?_____

_____

_____

_____

How could your approach be improved?_____

_____

_____

_____

What is one thing that you are willing to commit to in the next week to improve your sleep?_____

_____

There are negative consequences to our brain health when we look at a cell phone screen right before bed. Looking at screens causes the mind to activate instead of slowing down for sleep time. It also prevents the glial cells from healing and cleaning the body.[xix]

The product, Calm, is a highly absorbable form of magnesium that you can take before bed sprinkled in Yogi brand bedtime tea. When you're under stress, magnesium is the first mineral to be depleted. "Eboost" packets are an excellent energy drink alternative. (For more recommendations on eating/general wellness, go to "Free Talks" at GreenLightHeidi.com.)

Name an example of when you ate and/or drank something that made you feel bad and clogged your mind:_____

_____

How do you feel that eating affects optimal mental functioning?_____

_____

_____

Name one thing you'll do to improve your diet:_____

_____

_____

My overall goal for this chapter is to convey that the benefits of regular meditation are scientifically confirmed and that mindfulness practices (and the resulting improved coherent mind tip) are an essential component of optimal mental functioning, as well as resilience to stress.

In closing this chapter, it's important to mention how someone with a history of trauma cannot initially experience the benefits of mindfulness practices in the same way as someone without significant trauma. Let me try to explain. A person without significant trauma might find a gentle yoga class with pranayama (breathing exercises) stress-reducing. However, someone with trauma, say severe PTSD, could become hyper-aroused in that same situation and be triggered in a way that is basically the opposite of stress-reducing. This is why it is advised that someone new to meditation start with a body scan instead of simply sitting in silence or doing breathing exercises. Dr. Siegel has a free "Wheel of Awareness" body scan meditation on his website.[xx]

If you have experienced significant trauma (or you just want to understand it better), I highly recommend Bessel van der Kolk's book, "The Body Keeps the Score: Brain, Mind, and Body in the Healing of Trauma." This book outlines the importance of Eye Movement Desensitization and Reprocessing (EMDR), neurofeedback, and community improv as therapeutic modalities to treat trauma.

I did EMDR therapy with a trained counselor nine months after my husband passed away and was able to get my appetite back. (I mention this as a physical example of how the modality helped me.) EMDR helped me to process my emotions and move forward. I feel like the body grieves and my grief manifested by a loss of appetite in particular. If you are interested in learning more about EMDR or neurofeedback be sure to find a licensed and trained therapist.

1.

2.

3.

4.

5.

6.

7.

8.

9.

10.

8 INTEGRATED BRAIN TIP

"The human brain is a construction project in which genetics supplies the building blocks but social interaction largely determines how they are put together." –Daniel J. Siegel, M.D.

For the next few chapters of the book we will focus on the integrated brain tip of the Wellness Triangle. Before we think about this tip further, let's outline some brain basics and how the brain responds to stress.

THE BRAIN

The brain has lovingly been called "the most impenetrable treasure chest."[xxi] At 86 billion neurons and counting, I believe the brain is a miracle treasure chest.[xxii]

In the past, scientists thought that brain growth stopped by age 25. Modern neuroscience has shown that the ability of new nerves to form (neurogenesis) and to make new connections with each other (neuroplasticity) is possible throughout the human lifespan. Dr. Rudolph Tanzi of Harvard University confirms this by saying, "It's now known that the brain can form new axons and dendrites up to the last years of life, which gives us tremendous hope for preventing senility, for example, and preserving our mental capacity indefinitely."[xxiii]

All this new scientific understanding of brain health is great news for adults of any age. *Neuroplasticity and neurogenesis prove you can teach an old dog new tricks.* Here is one example:

Dr. Siegel describes an inspiring case study of a 93-year-old man who uses mindfulness techniques to grow and transform his brain. "As he approached his ninety-fourth birthday, Stuart sent me a note: 'I cannot tell you how much fun I am having. Life has new meaning now. Thank you.' I thank him for teaching me, for teaching all of us, how resilient our integrative brains can be."[xxiv]

So, modern research has demonstrated how neuroplasticity, neurogenesis, and our brain's resiliency can help us appreciate that we can literally alter our own minds in order to best deal with stress.

9 THE TRIUNE BRAIN

"Everything hinges on how you relate to your brain. By setting higher expectations, you enter a phase of higher functioning. One of the unique things about the human brain is that it can do only what it thinks it can do." --Deepak Chopra, M.D.

Neuroscientists have developed a model to describe our brains based on three parts which are referred to collectively to as the triune brain. The three parts of the triune brain are the brain stem, the limbic brain, and the prefrontal cortex.[xxv]

The brain stem is the stem-like part at the base of the brain; it is also known as the reptilian brain. In evolutionary terms it is the most ancient part of the brain and controls basic functions like breathing, heart rate, blood pressure, and swallowing.

The limbic brain, also called the limbic system, is

a collection of structures that operate by influencing the endocrine system and the autonomic (unconscious) nervous system. Think of the middle of the interior of your brain as the general location for the limbic brain. While we don't need to be able to name all the structures, you might have heard of the amygdala, the hypothalamus, and the hippocampus as parts of the limbic brain.

What's most important to know about the limbic brain is that your emotional life is largely housed here and it has a great deal to do with the formation of memories. The fight/flight/freeze mode of behavior originates in the limbic brain.

To complete the three elements of the triune brain is the prefrontal cortex, sometimes called the neocortex. This is the region of the frontal cortex, at the very front of the brain (located in your general forehead area) and is involved in problem solving and complex thought. Some functions of the prefrontal cortex include morality, intuition, higher reasoning, and fear modulation (the ability to unlearn a fear). The prefrontal cortex is basically the part of the brain that thinks about thinking. I'm asking you to use it to think through the concepts in this book and apply them in your life. Maybe take a moment and massage your forehead thanking your amazing prefrontal cortex!

10 THE BRAIN AND STRESS

"The mind uses the brain to create itself. As patterns of energy and information flow are passed among people within a culture and across generations, it is the mind that is shaping brain growth within our evolving human societies." --Daniel J. Siegel, M.D.

When you are experiencing stress, the limbic brain is firing (think, "fight, flight, freeze mode") and the prefrontal cortex is offline. (Remember: the prefrontal cortex is the part of the brain around the area of your forehead and is where executive functioning and higher reasoning occur and the limbic brain controls our instinctual reactions.)

This is the reason why counselors will teach hostile couples self-calming techniques when their interactions become too heated: their prefrontal cortexes are basically offline and consequently, they are not going to be capable of having much empathy and higher reasoning. One recent study shows that "routine daily stress shuts down the prefrontal cortex, the part of the brain responsible for decision making, correcting errors, and assessing situations."[xxvi]

Whenever you are feeling emotionally charged, agitated, or "on edge," I suggest practicing breath awareness, prayer, and/or self-calming techniques (HINT: this is when strengthening the coherent mind tip pays off). Mindfulness and breath awareness activities keep the body's stress response from taking over executive functioning. Note: there are many good and brief meditation videos for free on the internet.

Think about a time recently when you were under a lot of stress. How were you feeling?_____

_____

_____

Describe the situation here:_____

_____

_____

_____

_____

_____

_____

_____

What did you like about how you handled it?_____

_____

_____

_____

_____

What do you wish you had done better?_____

_____

_____

_____

_____

Consider the idea that we are never upset for the reason *we think* we are upset. Pretend that last sentence is 100% true and hypothesize some theories as to why you were actually upset about the stressful situation.

Theory#1 (why you were "actually" really stressed out):

_____

_____

_____

Theory#2:_____

_____

_____

Theory#3 (e.g., it was actually his/her hospitalization one month ago that wore me out, etc.)_____

_____

_____

Consider the next time you will be in crisis. What will you do now to set yourself up so that you are able to handle the stress better?_____

_____

_____

_____

_____

In America, we live in a culture that largely ignores prevention. Sayings like "a stitch in time saves nine" seem to go by the wayside in our busy schedules. Still, even in this overwhelming cultural climate, you can take action and plan ahead to help overcome stress.

Planning lets you have more space to focus on the *essential* instead of getting bogged down. This lets you deal with inevitable stressful situations that come up as a caregiver every day.

One great example of this is creating a durable power of attorney, a healthcare surrogate, and a living will. These documents ensure that IF something happens to you, you have a plan in place which protects your values and assets. Five Wishes is an excellent starting place. It was created by the lawyer for Mother Theresa and serves as a healthcare surrogate and living will in most States. *If you only complete one document, I recommend completing a power of attorney.* In the event that you become incapacitated (temporarily or permanently), this document states who can handle your affairs. Always consult with an attorney when creating legal documents.

11 BRAIN INTEGRATION

"Our brain's memory is altered by each revisiting of an experience."   --Dr. David A. Sousa

Now that we have explored the triune brain and the limbic brain vs. the prefrontal cortex, let's return to the brain integration tip of the Wellness Triangle. In the Wellness Triangle diagram, "brain integration" is defined as "having balance and quality in the physical integration between and inside the different parts of your brain."

Studies show that new challenges (learning a new musical instrument or language, even driving a different way to get from home to the doctor) help increase neurogenesis and neuroplasticity. There are online computer programs such as Lumosity or the Brain Fitness Centers of Florida that bill with insurance and help to strengthen your brain with exercises – this is like physical therapy for the brain.

Physical exercise where your heart rate increases, even walking, is fantastic for your brain health (as well as overall physical health). Exercise is one of the very few clinically proven methods to reduce the effects of stress and depression, and lab studies have shown that exercise can increase the rate of neurogenesis, even in aging.

See the diagram on the next page about the numerous benefits of exercise from the American College of Sports Medicine.

What do you do for regular exercise?_____

_____

_____

What was your attitude about exercise when you were a child? How does this influence/not influence your attitude and choice to exercise now?_____

_____

_____

What activity are you willing to commit to within the next week?_____

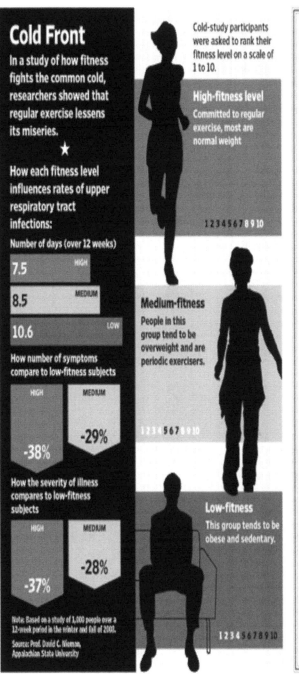

Cold Front

In a study of how fitness fights the common cold, researchers showed that regular exercise lessens its miseries.

★

How each fitness level influences rates of upper respiratory tract infections:

Number of days (over 12 weeks)

7.5 HIGH

8.5 MEDIUM

10.6 LOW

How number of symptoms compare to low-fitness subjects

HIGH MEDIUM

-38% -29%

How the severity of illness compares to low-fitness subjects

HIGH MEDIUM

-37% -28%

Note: Based on a study of 1,000 people over a 12-week period in the winter and fall of 2001.

Source: Prof. David C. Nieman, Appalachian State University

Cold-study participants were asked to rank their fitness level on a scale of 1 to 10.

High-fitness level
Committed to regular exercise, most are normal weight

1 2 3 4 5 6 7 8 9 10

Medium-fitness
People in this group tend to be overweight and are periodic exercisers.

1 2 3 4 5 6 7 8 9 10

Low-fitness
This group tends to be obese and sedentary.

1 2 3 4 5 6 7 8 9 10

Other studies show that exercise...

★ Lowers the risk of stroke by 27%.

★ Reduces the incidence of diabetes by approximately 50%.

★ Reduces the incidence of high-blood pressure by approximately 40%.

★ Can reduce mortality and the risk of recurrent breast cancer by approximately 50%.

★ Can lower the risk of colon cancer by over 60%.

★ Can reduce the risk of developing Alzheimer's disease by approximately 40%.

★ Can decrease depression as effectively as Prozac or behavioral therapy.

Source: American College of Sports Medicine

Wellness Triangle

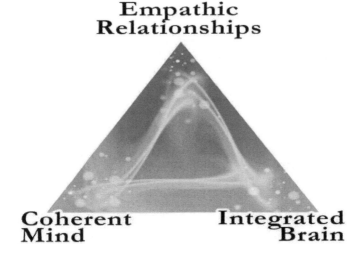

Empathic Relationships

Coherent Mind

Integrated Brain

<u>B</u>

<u>BRAIN INTEGRATION</u>

On a scale of one to ten, how do you rate your memory?_____(If you are concerned, please follow up with a neurologist. For a baseline, grab a timer and name as many animals as you can in one minute. Do this test once a year. If you name 14 or fewer animals, this indicates cognitive impairment.)_____

_____

Out of the ideas listed above that help improve brain integration (new challenges, exercise, and brain games/activities) write one new activity you are willing to try. When?_____

When you are under high levels of stress such as a crisis situation, what can you do to help remember that the limbic brain is firing and the prefrontal cortex (and higher reasoning) is offline? (I am asking this question for AFTER you've dealt with the initial mandatory concerns of the crisis.)_____

_____

_____

_____

Some of my suggestions for this question are having one of your close friends act as an "emergency buddy" you call that has also read this book and can help you, or having a visual reminder on the fridge, or a "safe zone" in your house where you can go to shut off your brain for a few minutes (or hours) while the fight/flight/freeze mode calms down, and simply reminding yourself that when you are extremely stressed out it's okay to say, "let me get back to you on that," if anyone wants you to make a complex decision that requires a fully functioning prefrontal cortex. If you *have to* make a complex decision (sometimes people will try to rush you when the decision can wait) remember this is when to call upon a trusted, high-quality relationship in your life to help you decide.

I believe the limbic brain vs. prefrontal cortex is one reason why someone who has just lost a spouse is encouraged to NOT make any major decisions for at least one year. The intensity of the grief clouds the functioning of the prefrontal cortex after the death (or any major trauma). Again, *every circumstance is different.* If you have been experiencing anticipatory grief as a caregiver, such as when a loved one is given a terminal diagnosis, the ability to make clear decisions after a loss might come back sooner. I decided to go back to graduate school for social work five months after my husband passed away. It took another nine months before I was attending classes, but personally, that decision and the following focus which was required to carry-through with it, was one of the smartest decisions I have ever made.[xxvii]

The social work program surrounded me with caring people, so that I felt connected (empathic relationships tip of the Wellness Triangle), and this gave my life meaning and purpose in the face of devastating loss. Meaning and purpose are vital parts of mental health. If you are weighed down with the responsibilities of caregiving, it is important for your brain integration to hold on tight to activities that make your life meaningful.

Personally, I went through a long phase while caregiving where I felt that life WAS meaningless. I had been full of positivity and very Pollyannish as a young adult and I needed to come to terms with the fact that life can feel extremely meaningless, especially in the face of devastating news. Studies show that successful grief resolution involves how we make meaning out of our circumstances. Grieving and grief resolution are parts of brain integration.

When someone dies, your memory of them is literally stored in the neural pathways in your brain. When you mourn their death, you are physically retracing those neural pathways. Deciding what the sadness "means" in the greater picture of your life is important to integrating those memories in your brain (as opposed to shelved away and denied). Dr. Siegel writes, *"When we block our awareness of feelings, they continue to affect us anyway. Research has shown repeatedly that even without conscious awareness, neural input from the internal world of body and emotion influences our reasoning and decision-making...in other words, you can run but you cannot hide.'*[xxviii]

Perhaps knowing that you cannot hide will help bring strength to your caregiving journey to embrace the gamut of emotions inherently involved with grief and anticipatory grief.

My experience with grief was that it was like cloudy weather - it would eventually pass - but I had to sit with it and feel it. Many times in my husband's final year and for the year after he died I only wanted to be alone in nature or with other widows/widowers. **I encourage the reader to embrace what you need without judgment in every phase of caregiving.** Confronting these emotions with an open mind encourages integration.

Remember the three tips of the Wellness Triangle (empathic relationships, coherent mind, and an integrated brain) and be aware that all three are vital for optimal mental health. Making consistent efforts to reduce your stress levels will not only make you a better caregiver, but it will ensure the likelihood of your good physical health far into the future.

11 THE RIVER OF BRAIN INTEGRATION

"As a species, we should take time every day to be thankful for this amazing organ buzzing away in our heads. Your brain not only transmits the world to you but essentially creates that world."
—Deepak Chopra, M.D. and Dr. Rudolph Tanzi

Now that you understand the three tips of the Wellness Triangle, we will use it as a metaphor for optimal mental health *in action* for caregivers.

Imagine the Wellness Triangle is like the steering wheel of a boat traveling down the River of Brain Integration. On each riverbank is either rigidity or chaos. You steer best down the river when you are **F**lexible, **A**daptable and **St**able (the F.A.St flow) down the River of Brain Integration. [xxxi]

If you don't have enough **F**lexibility, **A**daptability, and **St**ability in your life, you won't steer the boat well and will end up on the riverbank of either rigidity or chaos. For example, too much stability and not enough flexibility, ends up in rigidity. Too much flexibility and adaptability, and not enough stability, you end up in chaos. One example of this model is seen in dieting. At the beginning of a diet, there's usually a lot of rigidity around eating. The dieter is stuck on the riverbank of rigidity. When that can't be maintained, the dieter often starts binge eating, squarely landing on the opposite riverbank of chaos.[xxxii]

Draw a picture on the next page of your boat with the "Wellness Triangle" steering wheel flowing F.A.St down the River of Brain Integration. Be sure to include the two riverbanks. After you draw this picture, I suggest you skip the exercises on pages 63-64 and come back to them after you've read the entire chapter.

(The "F.A.St" and "rigidity/chaos" terms used in the above river analogy are based on extensive brain research. See the articles and books referenced in this chapter in the Index.)

Draw a Picture of You Steering a Boat
Down the River of Brain Integration:

Draw a picture of you **not** flowing F.A.Stly down the river. Let yourself wash ashore on one riverbank. Did you have too much flexibility or stability? What behaviors or thoughts slow you down?

Draw a picture of you flowing F.A.Stly down the river. Make a list of the thoughts that you are thinking and the activities that you are doing which cause you to keep a balance of flexibility, adaptability, and stability.

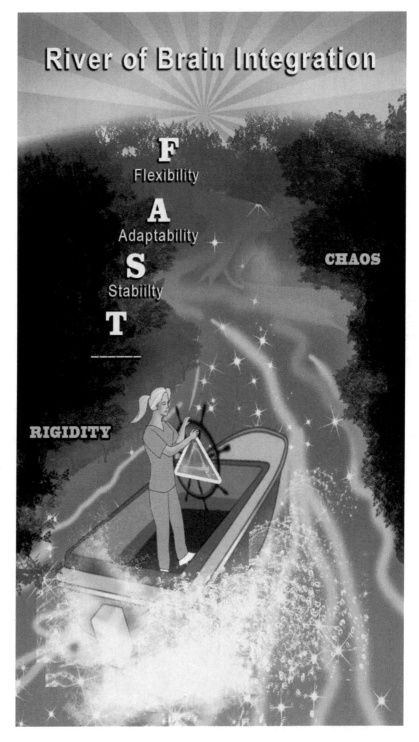

So how does cultivating a coherent mind, an integrated brain, and quality relationships help you flow F.A.St down the River of Brain Integration?

Before I can answer that question, we have to discuss your Super Highway.

THE SUPER HIGHWAY

Messages and thoughts in your brain are transmitted through neurons via electrical energy. This energy moves through fine processes called axons and dendrites. We now know that the axons and dendrites of your neurons are thicker and that more connections are made between them during development through childhood. These connections become part of your own make up and determine your responses to stress as your grow into adulthood.

We'll call your learned stress response from childhood your "Super Highway." When you are under stress, your brain will naturally trend toward whatever instinctive coping mechanisms you learned as a child. For example, if the family response to stress was eating whenever an argument erupted, you might find yourself eating when very stressed.

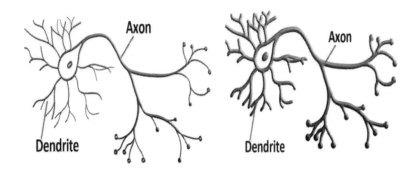

Thicker axons and dendrites from childhood

Awareness is the first step to successfully steering your boat down the River of Brain Integration. You are cultivating awareness every time you answer the questions proposed in this workbook.

What are some examples of your Super Highway? When you are under extreme stress, become triggered, and go "unconscious" with your actions what do you do?_____

_____

_____

_____

_____

_____

_____

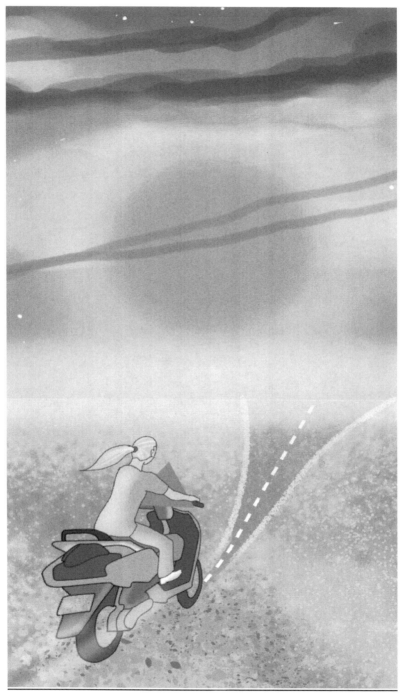

PAVING YOUR DIRT ROAD

PAVING YOUR DIRT ROAD

In chapter seven, we discussed how you can use mindfulness and awareness to shape and grow your own brain. In chapter eight, I outlined how neuroplasticity and neurogenesis are possible throughout life. I call this "Paving Your Dirt Road" and remind participants at workshops that it takes much longer to drive a motorcycle down a dirt road than it does a paved road.

Keeping in mind your Super Highway vs. Paving Your Dirt Road responses to stress, think about when you are more centered. Name an example of when you have responded more successfully and calmly in a stressful situation. Where were you and what was going on? _____

_____

_____

_____

_____

What about the above circumstance made you better able to respond instead of react? Had you taken some time for self-care recently? Was a supportive person with you?_____

_____

_____

What can you do now in your life to encourage the presence of whatever it is that you noted in the last question when your next stressful situation arises?_____

_____

_____

_____

Paving a Dirt Road and strengthening the three tips of the Wellness Triangle are keys to optimal mental health. Earlier I asked, "How does cultivating a coherent mind, an integrated brain, and quality relationships help you flow F.A.St down the River of Brain Integration?" The answer is that strengthening the three tips leads to a F.A.Ster flow down the river. Cultivating the three tips leads to increased capacity for flexibility, adaptability, and stability.

Focus on the parts of the Wellness Triangle that are weakest for you and take action to strengthen them. Also, if you tend toward the riverbank of chaos (by being too flexible and adaptable), practice cultivating stability. For clarification, "stability" here means maintaining a consistent mood and emotional expression as well as the ability to keep from getting unduly excited even in serious situations.

Two techniques that Dr. Siegel suggests that I love are "Name It to Tame It" and "A Feeling Is Not A Fact." Name it means you bring in the logical, left brain to name the emotion. The idea is that labeling it helps you detach a little from the intensity of the emotion. If you are very emotionally charged, naming the emotion is helpful, then stating: "this feeling is not a fact." This means just because we feel a particular emotion doesn't mean we *are* that emotion or that we have to react out of it. A good image is the emotion as a lake and sitting beside the lake instead of drowning in it!

If you tend toward rigidity, and have stability but not enough flexibility, practice pushing yourself beyond your comfort zone and increase your capacity to be flexible. In this context, flexibility means the ability to switch behavioral response according to the situation. Adaptability means being able to cope with adversity or danger without succumbing to basic emotions or impairment of your judgement. A useful technique is to pay attention to your peripheral vision and people's facial expressions. People who tend to be more logical, rigid, and left-brained have a harder time recognizing what emotion is on the face of the other. Ask a friend to support you in this and practice guessing his/her facial expressions.

Have compassion on yourself as you seek to grow and integrate. *Know that you will find yourself rushing down the Super Highway regardless of the strength of your resolve to change and grow.* Have compassion for your boat when it lands on the riverbank of rigidity or chaos. Lovingly dust it off, cry or scream if you need to, then put the boat back in the water as you begin to flow F.A.St down the River of Brain Integration again.

12 OPTIMAL SPIRITUAL HEALTH

"We think that the point is to pass the test or to overcome the problem, but the truth is that things don't really get solved. They come together and they fall apart." — Pema Chödrön

You made it! Most of this book has been about optimal *mental* health and much of the book's content required a lot of *cerebral* activity. In my opinion, no book on caregiving would be complete without bringing in a spiritual component. In this chapter addressing spirituality, we are moving from a two-dimensional triangle to a three-dimensional wellness pyramid.

From the beginning of this book, we examined the

positive nourishing aspects and the harder challenges encountered in the caregiving journey. Finding high-quality relationships where you receive love and attention is nourishing. Calming ever-racing thoughts and finding a quiet, centered mental space is nourishing. Learning to access the prefrontal cortex of the brain where intuition, morality, and higher reasoning occur is a more nourishing place to be than the fight/flight/freeze mode of the limbic brain.

The three tips of the Wellness Triangle are tangible and measurable concepts. We have examined these using evidence-based information and they are invaluable in helping you better understand the effects of stress on the mind and body. Now, we'll introduce the spiritual tip of the wellness pyramid, (see diagram on the next page).

I added the spiritual tip because caregiving taught me mostly about that which is unmeasurable and unseen. I learned how to relax (trust) more often when I was falling…and failing (in my eyes) as a caregiver. At one point I often repeated, "I forgive myself for mistakes made and things left undone."

What are some thoughts, prayers, or sayings that help to soothe you:_____

_____

_____

_____

_____

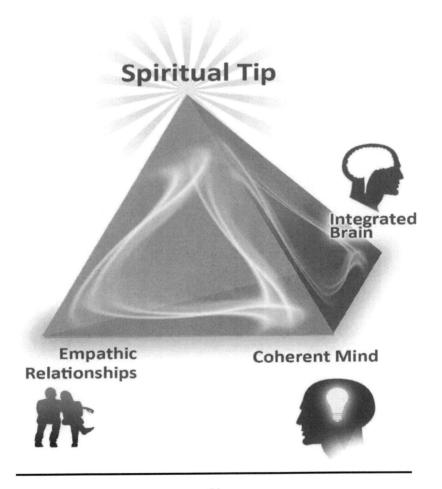

Spiritual Tip

Integrated Brain

Empathic Relationships

Coherent Mind

For me, part of the spiritual tip is related to nature. Nature gives unspoken, powerful nourishment. When I was a caregiver, Roger and I often spent time sitting quietly by the ocean or picnicking under live oak trees, especially as he became nonverbal. The silence and power inherent when we were in nature brought an experience of the spiritual to the fore at a time when I *most* needed it.

When I had a breakdown and had to move out of my home temporarily, this new space allowed me to increase the time that I spent engaging in a daily spiritual practice. In my experience, daily meditation, prayer, and chanting *always* helped calm my mind and emotions.

When Roger was under hospice and we had given up the search for more anti-cancer diets and natural remedies, all that was left was surrendering to God. Sometimes I could do this and sometimes I couldn't. From this experience, I would say there are no easy answers and it is up to each of us to decide.

The root of the word "decide" is "to slay," as in suicide or homicide. When we *decide* something, we are slaying all other possibilities by making one choice. As a caregiver, it took a long time for me to decide and establish clear answers. So, if you are in a state of not knowing "why" and unsure about what beliefs to slay or not slay about the nature of life, be gentle with yourself and find the love of people. **Other people's love kept me alive in my darkest times of grief.**

The spiritual tip is a difficult subject to write about, because people have vastly different religious and/or non-religious concepts. I don't intend to bog the reader down with any belief systems. **Still, it's *essential* to "point" to something deeper and more meaningful than optimal mental health alone.** So, here are some questions for you to think about the spiritual tip.

_____**Tip**

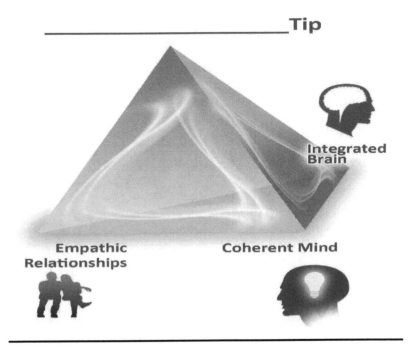

Reflecting on the wellness pyramid, I would name the top tip _____ and this is why:

_____

_____

_____

_____

How does the spiritual/_____ tip affect all other aspects of the wellness triangle? How does it affect your mind?_____

_____

_____

_____

How does the _____ tip affect/influence your brain?_____

_____

_____

How does the _____ tip influence your relationships?_____

_____

_____

Write about what makes your caregiving journey meaningful. What brings you hope on a bad day?_____

_____

_____

_____

_____

_____

_____

_____

_____

_____

_ How can you receive more spiritual nourishment?

_____

_____

_____

Write about where you go to get in touch with the _____ tip of the wellness pyramid:_____

_____

_____

_____

_____

Recall a time when you were under a lot of stress. Go ahead and pick another stressful situation that what you wrote earlier in the book when asked this question.

Describe the situation here:_____

_____

_____

_____

_____

_____

_____

_____

_____

What did you like about how you handled it?_____

_____

_____

_____

What do you wish you had done better?_____

_____

_____

_____

Consider the next time you will be in crisis as a caregiver. Keeping the spiritual/_____ tip in mind, what will you so now to set yourself up so that you are able to handle the stress better?_____

_____

_____

_____

There is a type of counseling is called "Solution Focused Therapy" where a client is asked what's known as the "Miracle Question." I'm going to end this book asking you this question. After you answer the question, reflect on your answer. My hope is that it brings you closer to achieving optimal mental and spiritual health.

Think about the biggest problem(s) you are facing right now. Write them here:_____

_____

_____

_____

_____

Let's say that you go to sleep tonight and when you wake up, these problems have been solved, like a miracle! What happens throughout the day which lets you know that the problem(s) have been solved? (Stay in a creative mindset as you answer this question, don't get bogged down with technicalities yet):_____

_____

_____

_____

_____

_____

_____

_____

_____

_____

_____

_____

_____

_____

_____

_____

_____

_____

_____

_____

Leave this book now and come back in five minutes.

Okay! Now that you are back from your break, reflect on your answer and write *a few things you can do* to move closer to this "miracle" solution:_____

_____

_____

_____

_____

_____

_____

In conclusion, I will say that *reading* about optimal mental and spiritual health and *experiencing* them are two very different things. Even though this is a book that you are reading, my aim is to help you fully experience optimal mental and spiritual health, to help you in your caregiving experience.

Compare the action of drinking a cool glass of water after a long day at the beach to the sensation of thirst and knowing in your mind that you need water. In this case, *drinking the water is far more refreshing.* It is the difference between using the word "try," as in, "I will try to meditate," and "practice," as in, "I practice a few minutes every day."

In the end, my hope is that we learn to "drink water" as caregivers (literally and figuratively!) and "practice" meditating and self-care instead of "trying to" do these things. Such acts are not only for the person we love, or only for us, but to improve the world we live and interact in.

AFFIRMATIONS FOR CAREGIVERS[xxxiii]

1. May I be honest with myself and others about my experience of suffering and loss.

2. May I find the inner resources to be present with my sorrow.

3. I forgive myself for mistakes made and things left undone.

4. May my love for others flow boundlessly.

5. May the power of loving-kindness sustain me.

6. May I find the inner resources to truly be able to give.

7. May I remain in peace and let go of expectations.

8. May I offer my care and presence unconditionally, knowing it may be met by gratitude, indifference, anger, or anguish.

9. May I offer love, knowing that I cannot control the course of life, suffering, or death.

10. May I see my limits compassionately, just as I view the suffering of others.

11. May I accept things as they are.

ABOUT THE AUTHOR

Heidi Crockett, LCSW, LMT, CMC, earned a BA in anthropology from Middlebury College and an MSW in social work from the University of Georgia. She completed post-graduate training from the University of Michigan's School of Social Work.

Heidi has worked as a social worker in hospital and community case management for over a decade and advocates for whole person health. She has published articles, appeared in radio interviews, and is a local and national conference speaker. Besides her professional experience, she was a caregiver for her husband until he passed due to his brain tumor in 2009.

INDEX

[i] From this booklet available online here: http://www.alz.org/downloads/facts_figures_2013.pdf, 38.

[ii] Shaw, W. S., et al. (1997)"Longitudinal analysis of multiple indicators of health decline among spousal caregivers." *Annals of Behavioral Medicine 19* (2), 107.

[iii] Siegel, D. (2010). *Mindsight: the New Science of Personal Transformation*. New York: Random House, 279.

[iv] Siegel, D. (2006). An Interpersonal Neurobiology Approach to Psychotherapy. *Psychiatric Annals, 36*(4), 248.

[v] In order to simplify things, when I write "neurobiology," I am technically referring to interpersonal neurobiology.

[vi] For those interested in knowing more about the Triangle of Well-Being, I recommend Dr. Siegel's book, *"Mindsight: the New Science of Personal Transformation."*

[vii] Gilbert, R. (1992). *Extraordinary Relationships*. New York: John Wiley & Sons, 3.

[viii] Floyd et al., 2007; Schwartz & Russek 1998; Floyd & Morman 2000

[xi] Resnick, S. (2012). *The Heart of Desire Keys to the Pleasures of Love*. New Jersey: John Wiley & Sons, Inc.,124.

[xii] http://www.strindbergandhelium.com/

[xiii] Siegel, D. (2010). *Mindsight: the New Science of Personal Transformation*. New York: Random House, 11.

[xiv] Kabat-Zinn, J. *Coming to Our Senses: Healing Ourselves and the World Through Mindfulness*. New York, NY: Hyperion; 2005.

[xv] Siegel, D. (2006). An Interpersonal Neurobiology Approach to Psychotherapy. *Psychiatric Annals, 36*(4), 250.

[xvi] Siegel, D. (2009). Mindful Awareness, Mindsight, and Neural Integration. *Humanistic Psychologist, 37*, 146.

[xvii] Williams, M., Teasdale, J., Segal, Z. and Kabat-Zinn, J. (2007). *The Mindful Way Through Depression: Freeing Yourself from Chronic Unhappiness*. New York: Guilford Press.

[xviii] Naiman, R. (2014). *Hush: A Book of Bedtime Contemplations*. Newmoon Media: Tucson, 8 and 3.

[xix] http://uk.businessinsider.com/smartphone-impact-brain-body-sleep-2015-2?r=US

[xx] http://www.drdansiegel.com/resources/wheel_of_awareness/

[xxi] Lewis T., Amini F. and Lannon R. (2000). *A General Theory of Love*. New York: Random House, 6.

[xxii] Azevedo, F., et al. "Equal numbers of neuronal and nonneuronal cells make the human brain an isometrically scaled-up primate brain." *J Comp Neurol*.513.5 (2009): 532-41.

[xxiii] Chopra, D. and Tanzi, R. (2013). *Super Brain: Unleashing the Explosive Power of Your Mind to Maximize Health, Happiness, and Spiritual Well-Being.* New York: Random House, 48.

[xxiv] Siegel, D. (2010). *Mindsight: the New Science of Personal Transformation.* New York: Random House, 119.

[xxv] The brain stem, limbic system, and neocortex are technically called "the reptilian complex, paleomammalian brain, and the neomammalian complex" in Paul D. MacLean's triune brain concept.

[xxvi] Chopra, D. and Tanzi, R. (2013). *Super Brain: Unleashing the Explosive Power of Your Mind to Maximize Health, Happiness, and Spiritual Well-Being.* New York: Random House, 108.

[xxvii] My personal philosophy is if I am feeling down and out at a certain point in my life, to go ahead and do something that will be good for my long-term well-being…what I've found is that at the bare minimum, I'm still feeling down doing what I've committed to doing, (e.g. going back to school,) but then I finish and I have increased self-confidence because I completed that task and increased social capital such as a degree, so that I have more job opportunities. Both these outcomes help improve the original "down and out" feeling.

[xxviii] Siegel, D. (2010). *Mindsight: the New Science of Personal Transformation.* New York: Random House, 125.

[xxxi] Siegel, D. (2010). *Mindsight: the New Science of Personal Transformation.* New York: Random House, 69-71. My analogy is adapted from his concepts and discussion of the "river of integration," "the riverbanks of rigidity and chaos," and "flexibility, adaptability, and stability".

[xxxii] "Diets do not lead to sustained weight loss or health benefits for the majority of people" from Mann, T., et al. (2007). Medicare's search for effective obesity treatments: Diets are not the answer. *American Psychologist,* 62(3), 220-233.

[xxxiii] Halifax, J. (2008). *Being with Dying.* Boston: Shambhala Publications. 100

Aquarius in Let The Sun Shine

Groovy Kind of Love

Come On People, Smile On Your Brother

Made in the USA
Middletown, DE
18 April 2015